Thank you to Karim

FORWARD

Confessions of a Habitual Rebel

How Tiny Habits Can Impact Your Life Negatively

Ever polished off a bag of chips mid-meeting while daydreaming about escaping to Tahiti? Scrolled through Instagram until your thumbs protested, only to realize you haven't moved from the couch since breakfast? Yeah, me too. Welcome to the hilarious, infuriating, and often energy-zapping world of our daily habits.

In my line of work – as a health coach and founder of Balanced Rebel – I've seen more hidden habit-demons than a haunted house convention. And guess what? They're not out there lurking in the shadows, they're nestled comfortably in our morning routines, evening rituals, and everything in between. These sneaky little saboteurs, disguised as harmless quirks, are quietly siphoning our energy, stealing our focus, and generally making life feel like a slow-motion obstacle course with extra sprinkles of stress.

But fear not! This book is your awakening secret weapon, a decoder ring for the language of habits. You'll meet the usual suspects – the sugar gremlins, the social media scroll-monsters, the procrastination procrastination-ers (yes, it's a thing!) – and we'll unveil their devious tactics. But more importantly, we'll equip you with tiny tweaks of awareness to disarm those bad boys and reclaim your energy, time, and sanity.

Think of this book as your personal rebel training camp, where we'll turn tiny adjustments into big life wins. We'll swap Netflix binges for real-life adventures, trade sugar highs for sustained energy, and turn social media envy into self-love anthems. Because let's face it, who needs a filter when you're radiating
inner sparkle?

So put on your rebel dancing shoes, and get ready to reclaim your life, one small habit at a time. Remember, it's not about becoming a productivity robot or a zen master – it's about feeling more alive, more energized, and more like the awesome, quirky, imperfect masterpiece you truly are. This is your invitation to rewrite your story, one tiny tweak at a time. Let's do this!

Onward to the revolution!

Rui da Silva, Founder and Head Rebel at Balanced Rebel

(P.S. Don't worry, I'm not judging the chip habit – those things are practically potato crack. We'll deal with that later.)

BALANCED|REBEL

BY
RUI
DA
SILVA

50 HABITS

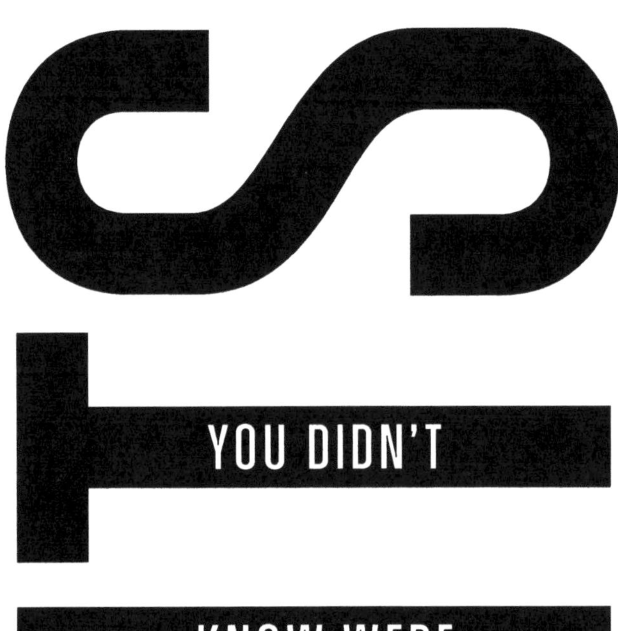

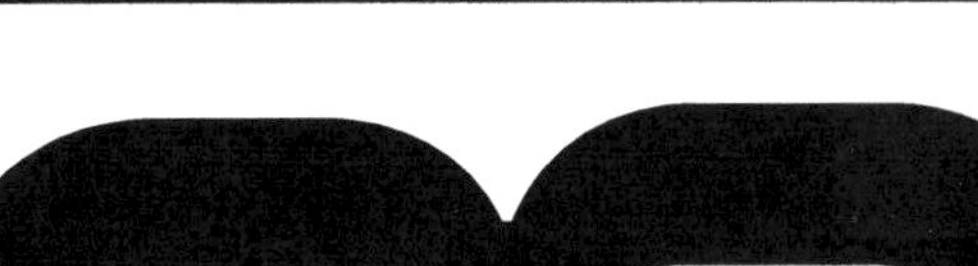

YOU DIDN'T

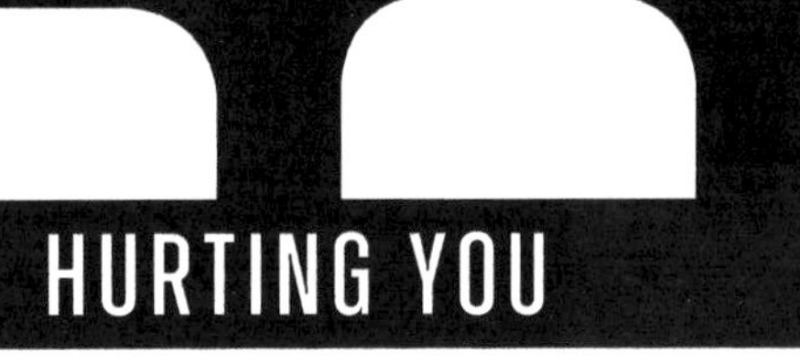

KNOW WERE

HURTING YOU

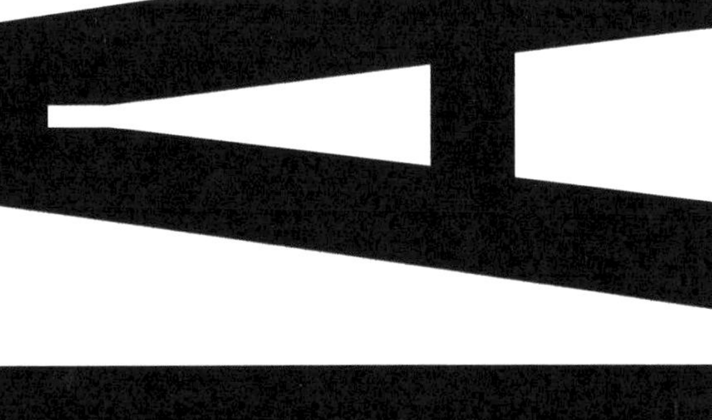

Title: 50 Habits That You Didn't Know Were Hurting You
Year of publication: 2024; Self-published
Founder and Head Health Coach of Balanced Rebel, online Health Coaching Company (balancedrebel.com)
Design by Hajer Ghareeb

HELPING INDIVIDUALS RECLAIM CONTROL OF THEIR LIFE ONE STEP AT A TIME

50 HABITS

#1

SCREEN TIME AS A STRESS RECOVER, AKA "RELAXATION" TECHNIQUE AFTER A BUSY/LONG DAY AT WORK

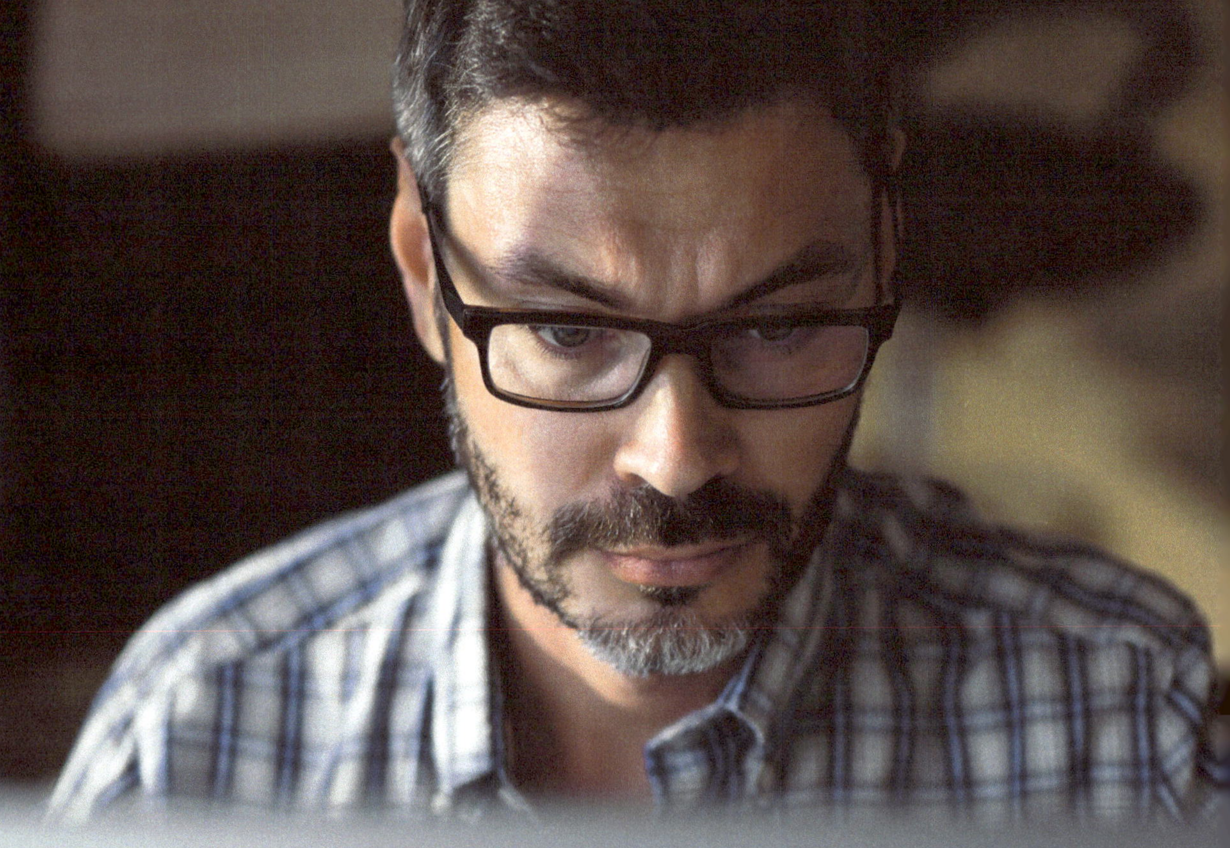

Engaging in enjoyable activities is certainly important, but it's also crucial to address the root causes of stress to prevent long-term buildup. Finding pleasure is great, but neglecting underlying stress might lead to bigger problems down the line.

#2

FREQUENTLY SAYING "I DON'T HAVE TIME"

When you utter the words "I don't have time", you are essentially conveying that the activity or task in question isn't a priority for you. It's true that we often fill our days with more tasks than time allows, rendering it impossible to accomplish everything we desire. That's precisely why, in our fast-paced lives, it's crucial to strategically plan and prioritize the essential, non-negotiable tasks that hold the potential to positively influence our lives.

#3

PROLONGED PERIODS OF NOT CONSUMING FOOD AND SKIPPING MID-DAY MEAL

Between juggling tasks and deadlines, meals can easily get pushed aside. But remember, food is our fuel! Skipping meals can lead to “reward seeking” later, making us crave sugary or processed options that might not leave us feeling our best.

#4

IGNORING THAT JOY IS THE FOUNDATION OF HAPPINESS

We often become overly fixated in the notion that happiness is attained through material possession (such as the perfect house, car or career), inadvertently overlooking the fact that a truly contented life hinges on the presence of joy. This personal sense of joy, whatever it may encompass for each individual, is a vital component of genuine happiness. It's essential to recognize that our well-being is intricately linked to happiness, or its absence, and in turn significantly imapacts our overall health.

#5

IGNORING THE SIGNS OF YOUR BODY

Every single day, your body communicates with you, sending out signals and messages that reveal its state of being. Yet, more often than not, these signals go unnoticed or worse, ignored. We exist in a society where the allure of quick fixes and instant relief often overshadows the deeper wisdom our bodies hold. So next time your body signals discomfort, don't silence it with a pill. Engage with it, listen to what it's trying to say.

#6

POOR COMMUNICATION IN YOUR RELATIONSHIPS

Whether in our professional endeavours or personal lives, we all engage in relationships that can potentially induce stress and anxiety. Practicing effective communication not only enables us to express our thoughts but also helps reduce the impact of repetitive and distressing thoughts in our minds.

#7

MINDLESS SNACKING

Many of us enjoy indulging in snacks during work hours or while watching T.V. However, regularly consuming unhealthy snacks leads to weight gain and unhealthy eating habits. Moreover, most of the time, these snacks are consumed out of boredom or in response to stress.

#8

USING THE WEEKEND TO RUNWAY FROM THE LIFE YOU HAVE RATHER THAN USING IT TO CELEBRATE THE LIFE YOU LIVE

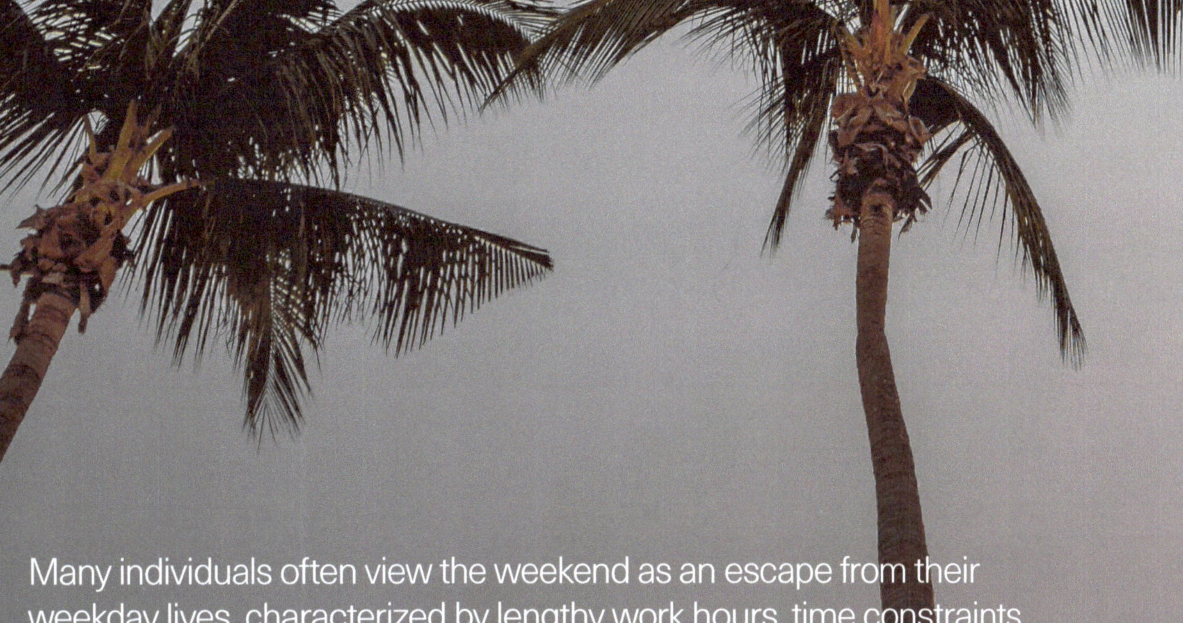

Many individuals often view the weekend as an escape from their weekday lives, characterized by lengthy work hours, time constraints, and overwhelming exhaustion. While it may initially seem enjoyable, this approach ultimately fails to provide the relaxation and rejuvenation needed. In reality, it can lead to increased stress and fatigue, setting the stage for a more exhausting and stressful week ahead.

#9

QUESTIONING THE IMPORTANCE OF SLEEP

During sleep, numerous crucial processes unfold. Your day doesn't truly commence upon waking; it commences the moment you retire to bed. The manner in which you sleep at night plays a pivotal role in shaping your performance and energy levels for the following day. The absence of a structured sleep routine and subpar sleep quality can profoundly influence both the quality and duration of your life.

#10

NOT SPENDING ENOUGH TIME EXPOSED TO DIRECT SUNLIGHT

Soak up the sun! Direct sunlight is your body's natural source of mood-boosting, Vitamin D, regulated sleep and supports overall well-being. Enjoy its benefits in moderation for a healthier, happier you!

#11

PROCRASTINATION

Procrastination is the practice of postponing tasks, often until the eleventh hour or even beyond their designated deadlines, despite being aware of the negative consequences. This avoidance stems from a desire to sidestep the stress and discomfort associated with the task, but this habit of last-minute delays can significantly increase stress levels, diminish performance, and result in emotional exhaustion.

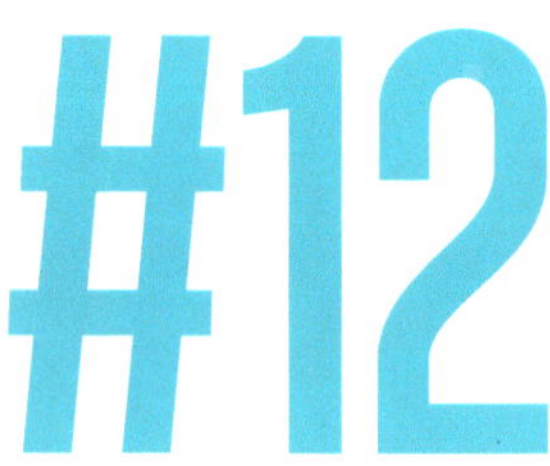

ALWAYS ON WORK CULTURE

Feeling constantly connected creates a sense of urgency and pressure, even when tasks are not genuinely urgent. This chronic stress takes a toll on your emotional and physical well-being, leading to anxiety, fatigue, and burnout.

#13

BELIEVING A "MAGIC PILL" OR INSTANT SOLUTIONS WILL BE SUSTAINABLE WITHOUT CHANGING ANY HABITS

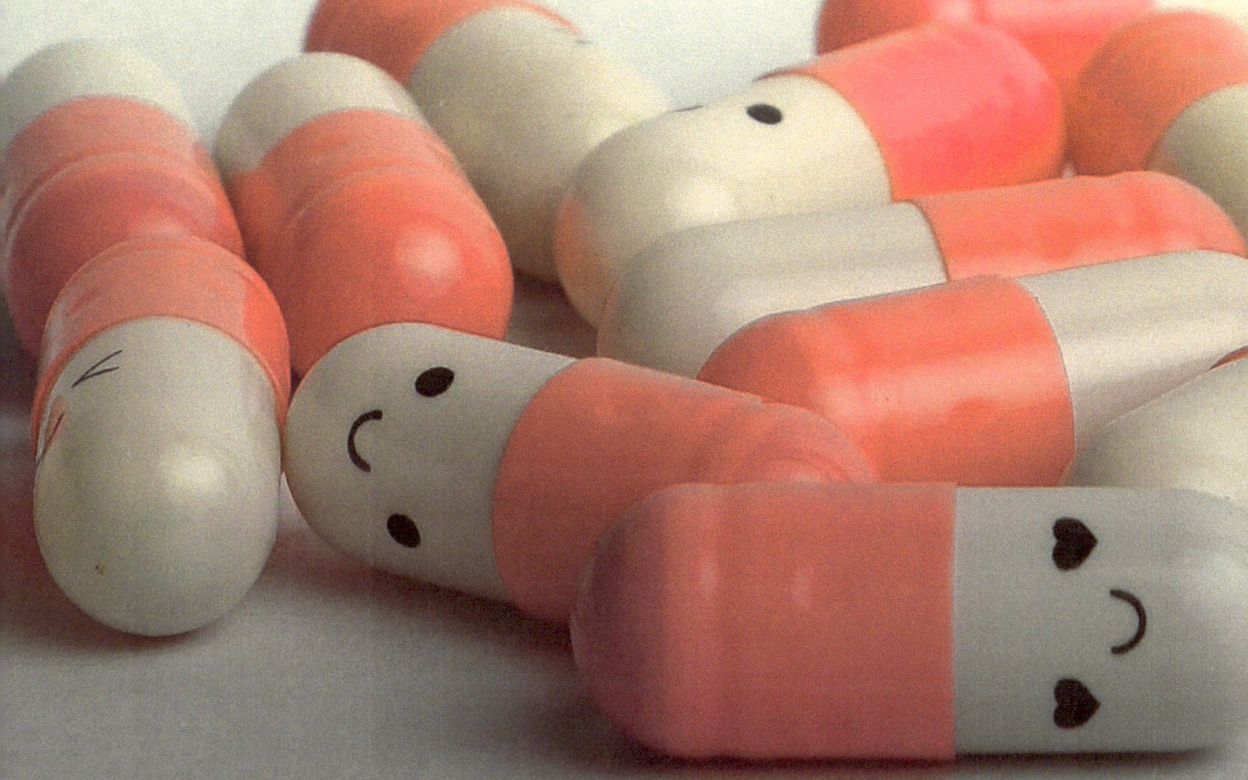

"Magic pills" or quick-fix solutions that promise to dramatically change one's life often don't work on the mid to long run for several reasons:

- Complexity of life
- What works for one person may not work for another?
- Unrealistic expectations
- They may provide short-term results but fail to produce lasting transformations.

#14

IGNORING THE SIGNS OF MENTAL FATIGUE

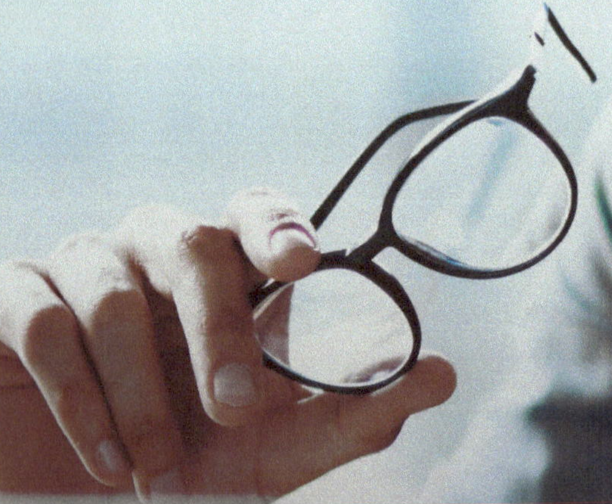

Ignoring the signs of mental fatigue can have serious consequences for your overall well-being, productivity, and even your physical health:

- Reduced productivity
- Physical health implications
- Emotional impact
- Decreased cognitive performance
- Impaired decision-making
- Risk of burnout
- Decreased work-life balance

#15

NOT DRINKING ENOUGH WATER

99% of your sweat is water, allowing your body to cool down and release toxins through perspiration. Adequate water intake ensures efficient sweating and prevents dehydration.

95% of urine is water, flushing out waste products and toxins from.

75% of the brain is made of water and it has no ability to store any of [illegible] carry out every conscious function.

#16

FREQUENTLY REVIEWING EMAILS OR WORK-RELATED MATTERS BEFORE BEDTIME

While work is undoubtedly important, prioritizing high-quality sleep is even more crucial. Winding down before bedtime is essential for fostering restful sleep. It's advisable to avoid engaging in activities that can excessively stimulate your mind before retiring for the night. Remember, insufficient sleep leads to reduced energy levels, and diminished energy translates to lower performance the following day.

#17

NEGLECTING SHORT BREAKS DURING WORKING HOURS

Many people assume that if they work continuously, the more content and high-quality work they'll produce. However, this belief is mistaken. Taking strategic breaks and moving your body can boost productivity. Breaks can increase your heart rate, stimulate blood circulation, and deliver more nutrients and oxygen to the brain. So, by incorporating breaks, you not only reduce stress but also enhance your cognitive processes.

#18

MULTITASKING

Multitasking, often seen as a way to increase productivity, can indeed have a negative impact on your health and well-being. When multitasking, the brain has to divide the available resources (oxygen, nutrients and glucose) to complete the tasks in hand leading to:

- Increased stress
- Reduced focus
- Impaired memory
- Decreased efficiency
- Increased errors
- Exhaustion
- Sleep disruption

#19

OVERCONSUMPTION OF SUGAR

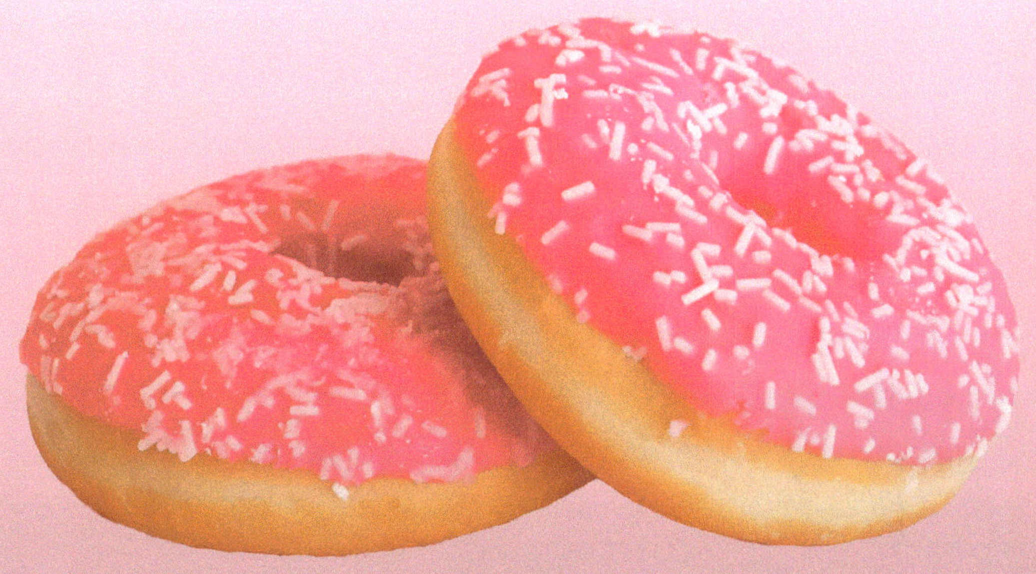

While indulging in treats occasionally is fine, overdoing sugary processed foods and beverages carries hefty costs beyond weight gain and diabetes. Here's why being mindful of your sugar intake can benefit your health, your wallet, and even your negotiation skills:
Energy dips: Sugar highs are followed by crashes, impacting your focus, productivity, and mood, especially during crucial negotiations.
Brain fog and fatigue: High sugar intake can decrease your cognitive function, alertness, and ability to think clearly, impairing your negotiation skills.

#20

EXCESSIVE SCREEN TIME OVER THE WEEKEND

The weekend is your chance to connect with yourself and the others. Don't let excessive screen time dull your mind and disconnect you from all the weekend's opportunities.

#21

POOR ERGONOMICS

Incorrect desk setups and poor ergonomics practices can lead to musculoskeletal issues, such has back pain and neck pain.

#22

STRESSFUL COMMUTES

A long and stressful commute can contribute to elevated stress levels and negatively affects mental health. Here are 3 strategies to help alleviate stress during your commute:

- Mindful breathing and relaxation techniques
- Transform the commute into an opportunity to walk more
- Listen to something relaxing and interesting instead of starting work calls
- Walk more if you can

#23

CONSUMING MORE CALORIES THAN NUTRIENTS

Consuming excess calories without essential nutrients can lead to weight gain, increasing the risk of obesity-related issues. Nutrient deficiencies can weaken the immune system and impair overall bodily functions. High-calorie, low-nutrient diets contributes to chronic diseases and inflammation. Prioritizing nutrient-rich foods is crucial for long-term health and well-being.

#24

THE BELIEF THAT "LOW FAT = HEALTHY EATING" IS TRUE

The food industry often paints "low fat" as synonymous with "healthy," but the reality is more complex. While minimizing fat intake can be beneficial, many manufacturers simply replace removed fats with sugars and refined carbohydrates to maintain palatability. This substitution, unfortunately, creates hidden health concerns.

Reading beyond the "low fat" label is crucial for making informed choices. Prioritize whole, unprocessed foods and healthy fats from sources like nuts, avocados, and olive oil. Don't let misleading marketing practices dictate your health.

#25

LIMITING BELIEF SYSTEMS

Limiting belief systems like "I'm too old", "too tired", or "my best days are gone" can bring stress, self-doubt, and health challenges. When you think "this is the only way", you are limiting your potential.

#26

REWARD STRATEGIES

Reward strategies (food, drinking, screen time, etc.), if misaligned or not well-balanced, can negatively impact your health for several reasons:

- Unhealthy choices
- Emotional eating
- Unsustainable habits
- Stress and guilt
- Short-term focus
- Financial impact

#27

DEMONIZING FOODS

The issue isn't the foods themselves; its our relationship with and how we consume them that truly matters. Blaming nutrients won't enhance your well-being; nutrients serve specific purposes, and embracing nutrient diversity is the cornerstone of a healthy life.

#28

BINGE-WATCHING TV

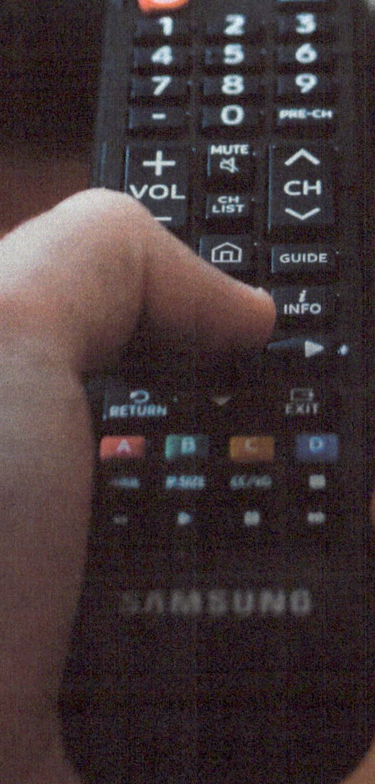

While spending extended hours in front of the TV can be a tempting escape from our busy weekday's lives, relying solely on this strategy for stress relief and "me-time" may not be conducive to long-term well-being. It can foster a sedentary lifestyle and disrupt your sleep patterns.

#29

IRREGULAR SLEEP PATTERNS

Staying up late and waking up at irregular hours can disrupt your sleep schedule and affect your sleep quality which impacts your energy and performance.

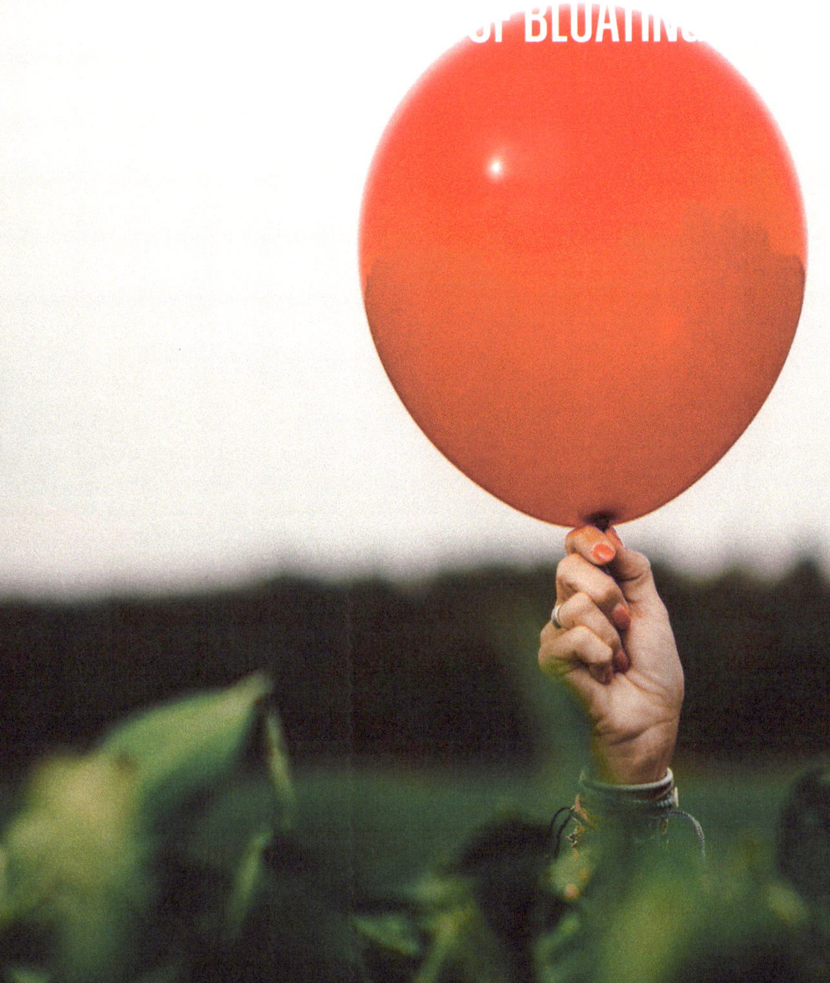

Experiencing bloating after a meal may signal an underlying issue. It's essential to recognize that bloating goes beyond mere discomfort, it can impact your life significantly. From undermining your confidence to affecting your daily routines, addressing bloating is a crucial step towards a happier healthier you.

Avoiding movement = risky business. Steering clear of movement not only impacts your physical health but can also affect your mental well-being. It's time to stand up, step out, and get those muscles moving for a healthier happier you!

#32

THINKING THAT CATCHING UP WITH SLEEP DURING THE WEEKEND WILL RESOLVE ACCUMULATED FATIGUE

Sure, those extra weekend snoozes might feel like a recharge, but here's the truth: its not the ultimate fix for accumulated fatigue. Consistent, quality sleep throughout the week is the real game-changer.

#33

OVERWORKING

Engaging in excessive work hours leads to burnout and increased stress.

#34

LACK OF SELF-COMPASSION

Mistakes are an inevitable part of being human. While we cant alter the past, accepting out failures without being too hard on ourselves is key. Emotional stress is real, and embracing self-compassion helps manage stress more effectively.

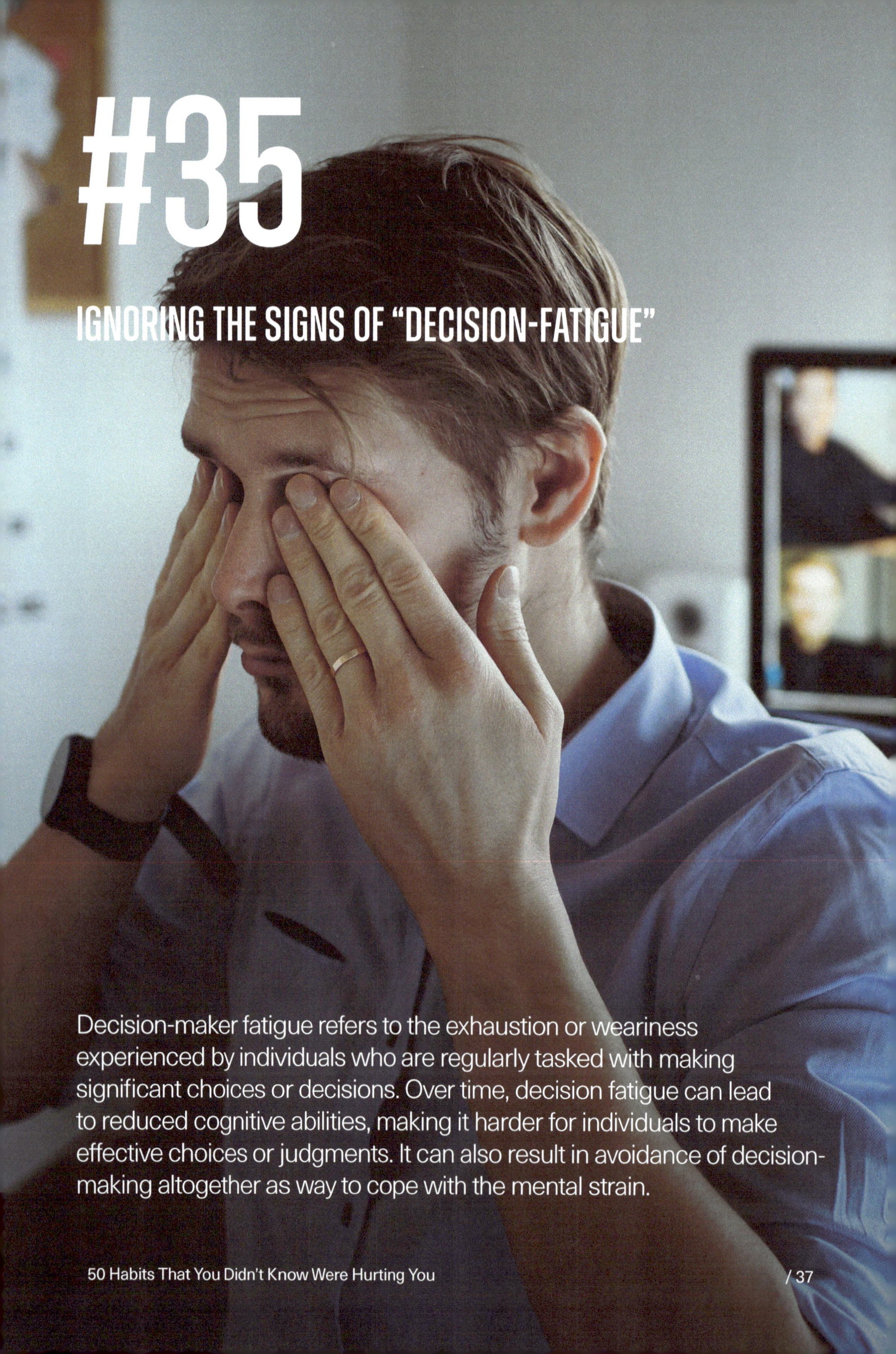

#35

IGNORING THE SIGNS OF "DECISION-FATIGUE"

Decision-maker fatigue refers to the exhaustion or weariness experienced by individuals who are regularly tasked with making significant choices or decisions. Over time, decision fatigue can lead to reduced cognitive abilities, making it harder for individuals to make effective choices or judgments. It can also result in avoidance of decision-making altogether as way to cope with the mental strain.

#36

BEING IMPATIENT WHEN COMMUTING

Being impatient while commuting can lead to various negative outcomes. Overall, being impatient during commuting not only affects personal well-being but can also impact the safety and experience of others on the road. Practicing patience can contribute to a more relaxed commuting experience for everyone.

#37

IGNORING THE SIGNS OF TRAVEL FATIGUE

Travel fatigue refers to the physical and mental exhaustion experienced during or after a journey. It's a result of extended periods of travel, time zone changes (jet lag), disrupted sleep patterns. Common symptoms of travel fatigue include tiredness, irritability, difficulty concentrating, headaches, disrupted sleep, muscle aches, and digestive issues. Factors such as long flights, extensive driving, or packed itineraries can intensify these symptoms.

#38

We have never been so connected and yet so lonely. Loneliness is a complex emotional state characterized by feelings of emptiness, isolation, or disconnection from others. Overall, loneliness impacts various facets of health, both mental and physical, emphasizing the importance of fostering meaningful connections and a supportive social network to maintain overall well-being.

#39

DRINKING LESS WATER IN THE WINTER

The colder weather makes us less inclined to drink fluids, but dehydration can become a serious issue in winter. Dehydration can lead to fatigue, headaches and impaired cognitive function. Aim to drink plenty of water throughout the day, even if you don't feel thirsty.

#40

[illegible]

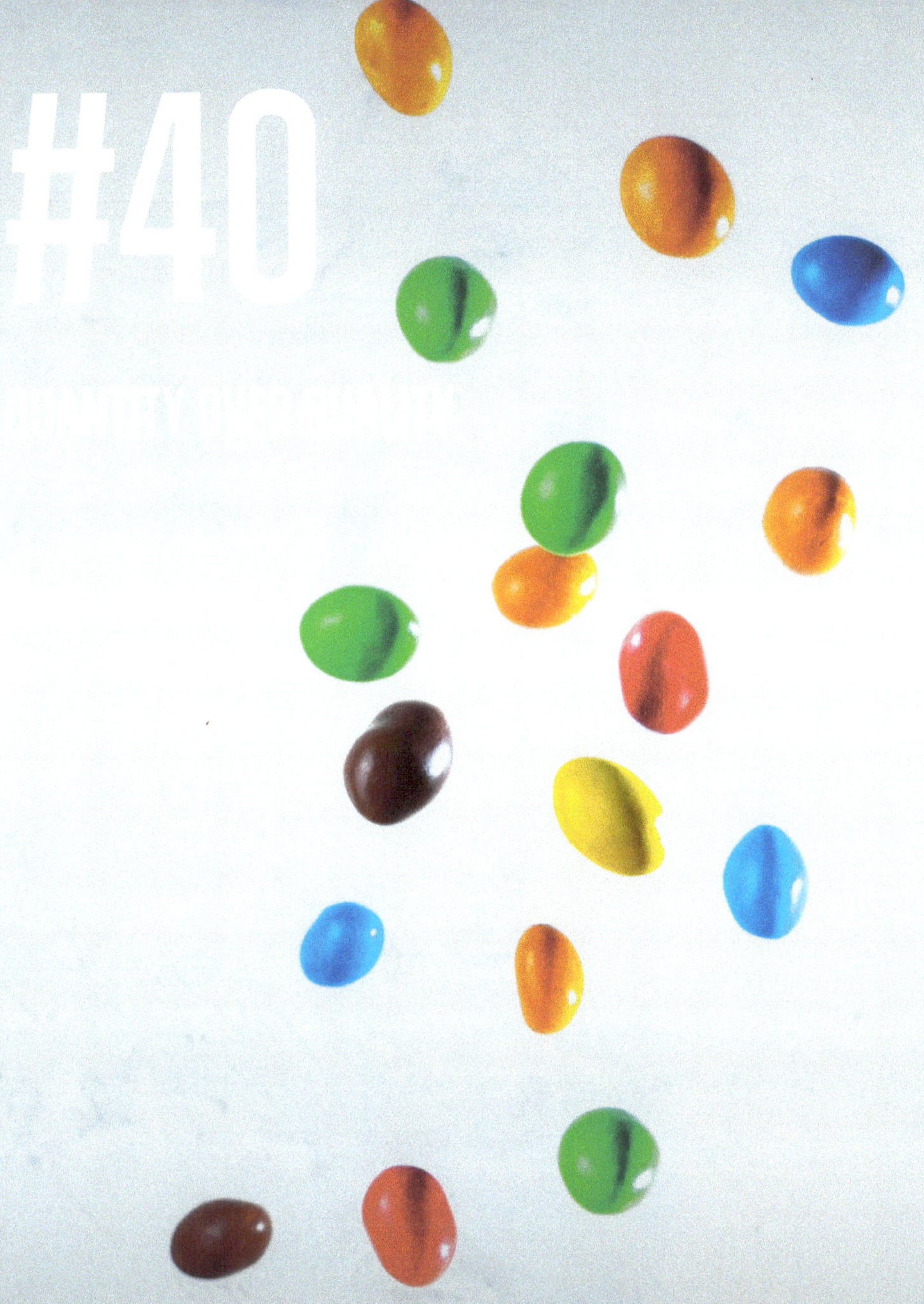

We often fall into the trap of believing that working longer hours leads to better work performance. Our time is finite, a precious resource that cannot be replenished. When we overstay at the workplace, we inadvertently steal time from other essential aspects of our lives, such as personal relationships, physical well-being, or pursuing personal interests. This imbalance can lead to burnout, reduced productivity, and an overall diminished quality of life.

#41

LETTING TECHNOLOGY USE YOU

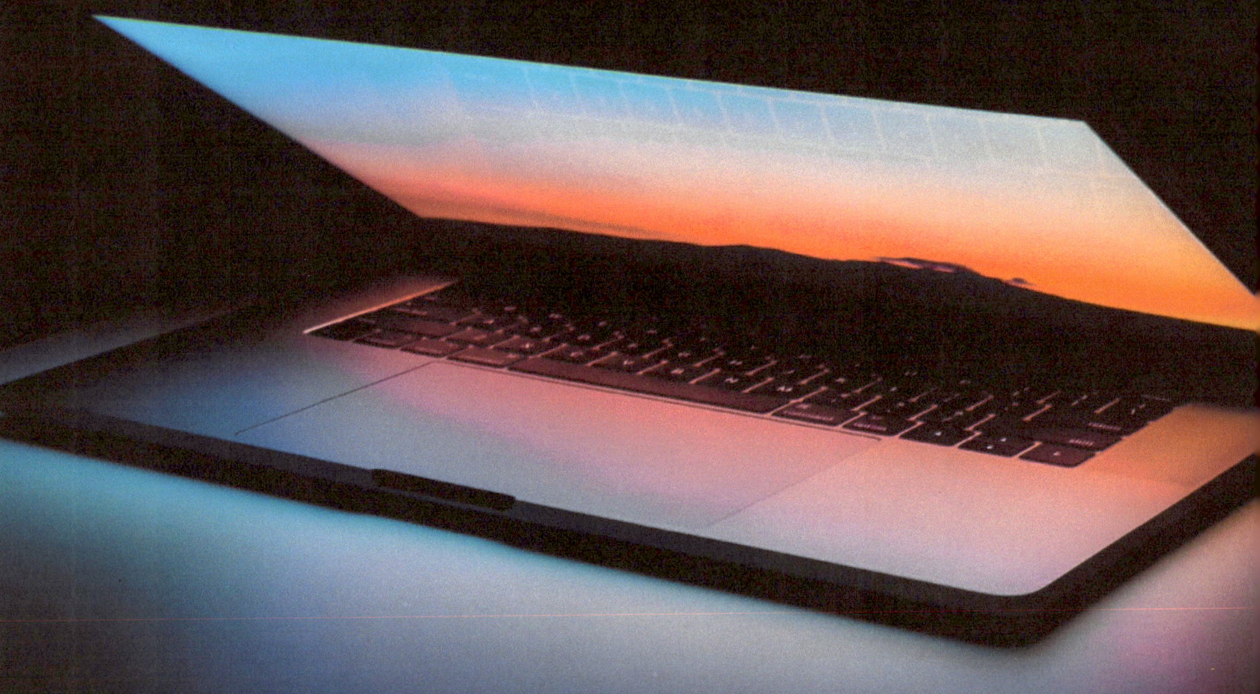

While technology can be inmensely helpful, its crucial to maintain control over it, rather than letting it control us. When technology becomes the master, it can lead to several negative consequences:

- Reduced productivity
- Eroding well-being, depression and feelings of inadequacy
- Limited creativity
- Diminished relationships

#42

DIETS OR FOOD RESTRICTIONS DURING HOLIDAY SEASON

Unless specifically advised by a doctor for health reasons, its crucial to embrace the holiday season to the fullest. Life is brimming with emotional and social occasions that deserve to be cherished to the fullest. While there are ample days in the year to focus on changing eating habits, this season is for indulgence, celebration, and savouring every moment. So, eat, indulge, and celebrate the joy of the season.

#43

TENSE FAMILY DYNAMICS

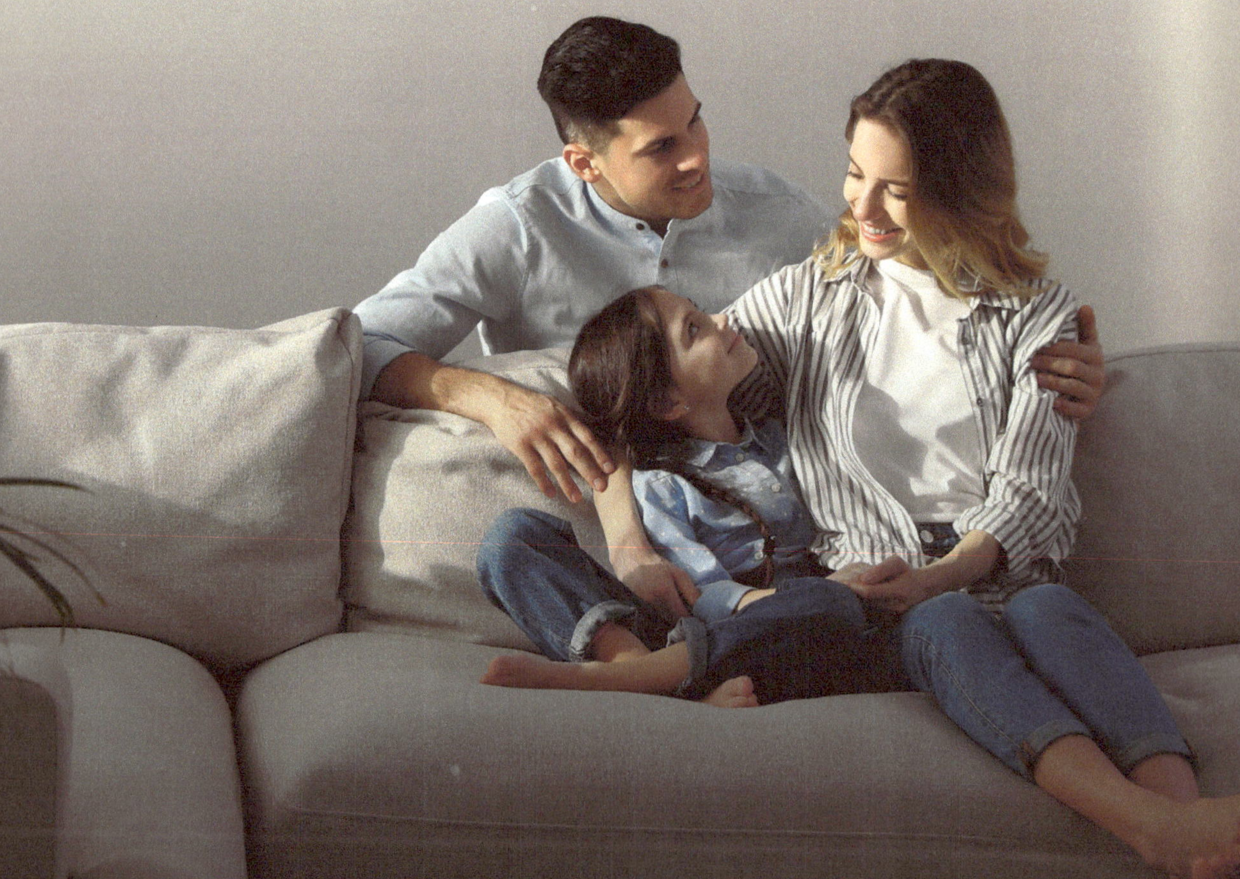

Tension within families, conflicts, or difficult relationships can be magnified during the holidays, causing stress and anxiety.

#44

SETTING GENERIC GOALS

Generic goals can impact your life negatively because they lack specificity and direction. When goals are too broad or vague, it becomes harder to create actionable steps or measure progress. This can lead to a lack of motivation, procrastination, and a sense of aimlessness, making it challenging to achieve meaningful results.

#45

NEGATIVE OUTLOOK ON THE WORLD

Overconsumption of negative news might create a pessimistic worldview, making individuals believe the world is more dangerous or negative than it actually is.

#46

LACK OF PRIORITY MANAGEMENT

Prioritization helps distinguish between urgent and important tasks. Without prioritizing, you night end up focussing on tasks that seem pressing but are not necessarily significant.

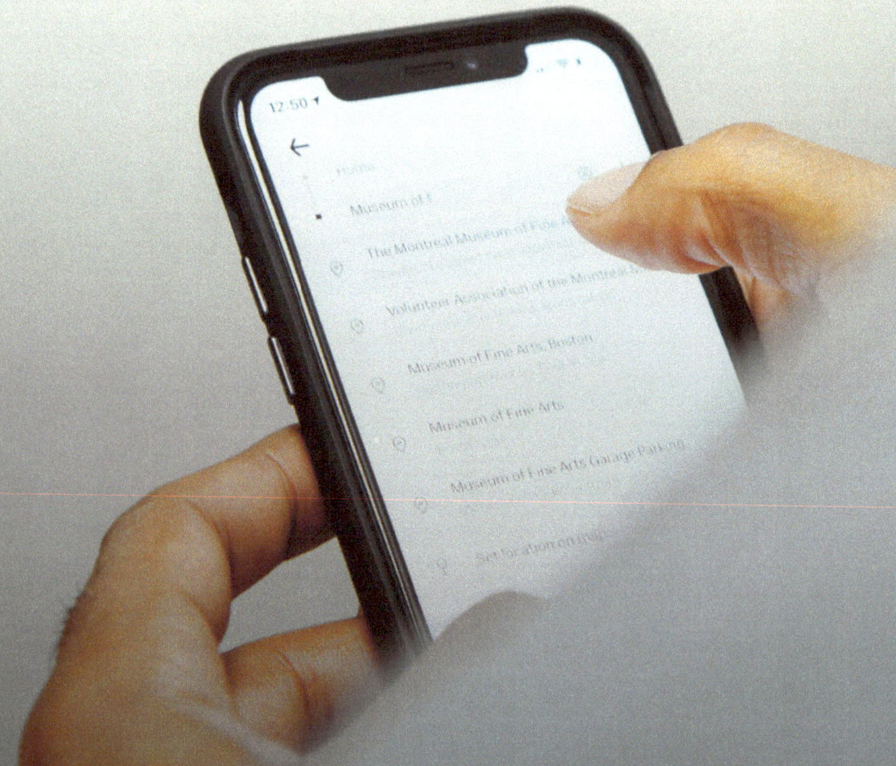

Mindlessly scrolling through negative news and social content feeds anxiety, negativity, and can disrupt sleep. Set time limits and curate your online spaces for more positive and inspiring content.

#48

EMOTIONAL EATING

Turning to food for comfort or emotional relief, known as emotional eating, can feel good in the moment, but it can have negative impacts on your health in the long run. Here's why:

- Nutritional imbalance
- Weight gain and chronic diseases
- Disrupted digestion
- Unsustainable cycle

Remember, fuelling your body with nutritious choices and addressing emotional wellbeing holistically leads to a healthier and happier you.

#49

PHONE PHANTOMS

Constantly checking your phone, even for unimportant notifications, can fragment your attention, disrupt conversations, and create a dependence on digital stimulation. Practice mindful breaks from your phone to be more present in your surroundings.

#50

PERFECTIONISM PANIC

Striving for perfection in everything can lead to procrastination, anxiety, and even burnout. Embrace progress over perfection, learn from mistakes, and focus on doing your best, not being the best.

BONUS
5 TIPS TO HELP YOU ON YOUR WEIGHT LOSS JOURNEY

Recently I had to have surgery which meant I couldn't exercise normally, turning my own health routine into a challenge. I felt like I was fighting an uphill battle against the scale. But as soon as I recovered, I put these 5 simple steps into action – and guess what? My pre-surgery weight was back before I knew it! I'm not talking about magic tricks, just smart tweaks that fueled my recovery. Making healthy choices feel effortless. Let's ditch the post-surgery blues and get you back to feeling amazing, inside and out!

#1

INTERMITTENT FASTING

I've been practicing a 16/8 intermittent fasting schedule (eating window from 12pm to 8pm) for the past 15 years. However, as a certified health coach, it's important for me to emphasize that starting any dietary change, including intermittent fasting, requires consulting a healthcare professional first.

While my personal experience has led to:
Improved blood sugar regulation: This is a potential benefit of intermittent fasting, but individual results can vary significantly. A healthcare professional can assess your individual needs and health status to determine if this approach is safe and appropriate for you.
Reduced digestive strain (potentially): Similar to blood sugar regulation, this is a potential benefit, but individual experiences differ. Consulting with a healthcare professional is crucial before making any significant dietary changes.
Establishing a healthier eating routine (for me): Finding a consistent eating pattern can be helpful for some, but it's crucial to approach it safely and with proper guidance.

Remember: My personal experience is just that, not medical advice. Intermittent fasting can have potential risks and isn't suitable for everyone. Always consult with a healthcare professional before making any changes to your diet or lifestyle, especially if you have any underlying health conditions.

#2

THE 80:20 RULE

Ditch the deprivation, embrace intention! I believe in making food choices that empower me, not restrict me. The 80/20 rule helps me prioritize whole, energizing foods 80% of the time. The remaining 20%? It's all about enjoying life and connecting with others through food. Energetic eating isn't about tasteless plates, it's about consciously choosing nutrient-rich options that build a stronger, happier you.

#3

MOVING THE BODY DAILY

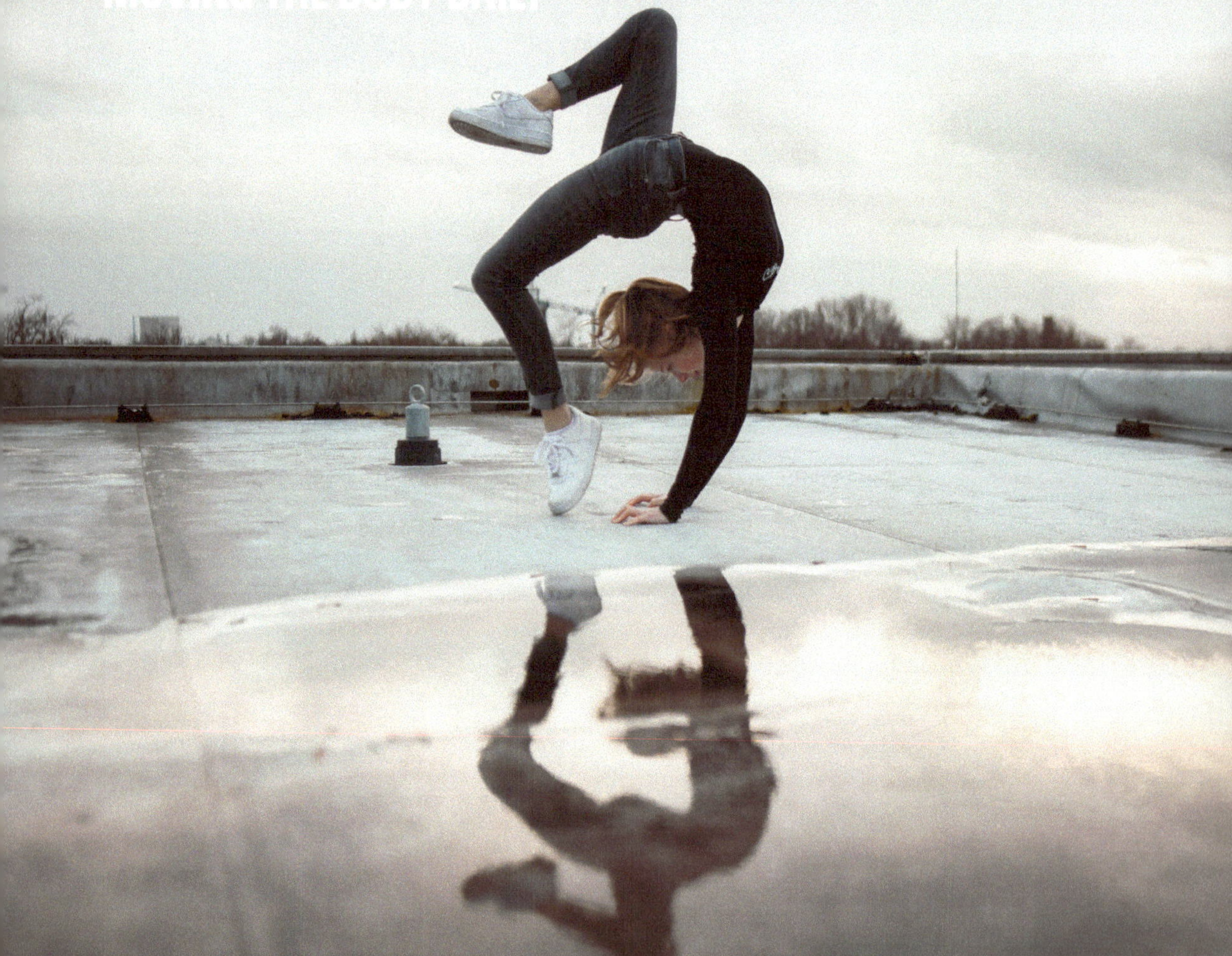

The human body thrives on movement. Exercise or simply staying active contributes to burning calories, lowering blood sugar levels, managing stress and anxiety, and fostering better sleep. Remember, the more you move, the more calories you burn, leading to a healthier, more energized you.

#4

SLEEP (7-9H DAILY)

Not prioritizing rest and recharging can lead to lower energy levels. When energy is low, decision-making abilities can diminish, making it harder to choose what's best for you. Your brain may crave rewards or sugary, high calorie foods in search of quick energy boost.

#5

IDENTITY

Achieving sustainable weight loss involves adopting a new identity – deciding who you aspire to be and identifying the habits that need transformation to reach that goal. Consider the analogy of a woman discovering she is pregnant; she swiftly embraces a new identity and adjusts habits seamlessly. Similarly, reshaping your identity and habits is pivotal in a lasting weight loss journey.

ABOUT THE AUTHOR

Rui da Silva is an expert coach in stress management, fatigue, sleep & recovery with a proven track record of transforming and enriching people's lives globally.

Known as Kootshi, he is the founder and head coach of Balanced Rebel, a health coaching company (balancedrebel.com).

With over two decades of excelling as a regional director for satellite companies worldwide, Rui possesses an in-depth understanding of the immense pressures placed on professional executives. He's acutely aware of the toll that constant travel, multi-million-dollar targets, and other stressors can exact on individuals striving to maintain a balance between their professional and personal lives.

Balanced Rebel was established as a holistic health coaching company to be a guiding light for busy professionals facing life's myriad challenges, providing them with the tools to improve their energy levels and to reclaim their lives on their own terms. Rui's mission is to unlock their greatest potential for success, one step at a time.

Rui, AKA "Kootshi" was named as one of the "Top 5 Coaches To Look Out For In 2022" by Entrepreneurs Herald, and in 2023 is the winner of the Holistic Health Coach of the Year by Corporate Live Wire. In 2024 Kootshi and Balanced Rebel have been nominated as health and wellness influencer of the year on the Global Health awards.

THANK YOU FOR READING

www.ingramcontent.com/pod-product-compliance
Lightning Source LLC
LaVergne TN
LVHW071152160826
845679LV00003B/636

* 9 7 8 9 4 0 3 7 2 3 8 0 8 *